VEGAN COOKBOOK FOR BEGINNERS

Quick & Easy Ketogenic Vegan Recipes that Anyone Can Cook at home

© Copyright 2021 - All rights reserved.

The content contained within this book may not be reproduced, duplicated or transmitted without direct written permission from the author or the publisher.

Under no circumstances will any blame or legal responsibility be held against the publisher, or author, for any damages, reparation, or monetary loss due to the information contained within this book. Either directly or indirectly.

Legal Notice:

This book is copyright protected. This book is only for personal use. You cannot amend, distribute, sell, use, quote or paraphrase any part, or the content within this book, without the consent of the author or publisher.

Disclaimer Notice:

Please note the information contained within this document is for educational and entertainment purposes only. All effort has been executed to present accurate, up to date, and reliable, complete information. No warranties of any kind are declared or implied. Readers acknowledge that the author is not engaging in the rendering of legal, financial, medical or professional advice. The content within this book has been derived from various sources. Please consult a licensed professional before attempting any techniques outlined in this book.

By reading this document, the reader agrees that under no circumstances is the author responsible for any losses, direct or indirect, which are incurred as a result of the use of information contained within this document, including, but not limited to, — errors, omissions, or inaccuracies.

Sommario

INTRODUCTION 7
VEGAN RECIPES 9
CAULIFLOWER BIBIMBAP 9
ROASTED BOK CHOY 13
VEGAN SHAKSHUKA 15
REFRIGERATED VEGETABLE SALAD 17
GINGER, SESAME, WALNUT AND HEMP SEED LETTUCE WRAPS 19
ROASTED PEPPERS AND ONIONS 21
CURRY PUMPKIN SOUP 23
TOFU PERFECT BAKED CRISPY 25
KETO CAULIFLOWER STUFFING 27
KETO VEGAN PIZZA STICKS 29
ZUCCHINI NOODLES WITH AVOCADO SAUCE 31
VEGAN TOFU BUFFALO WINGS 33
CAULIFLOWER RICE PILAF WITH HEMP SEED 36
GRILLED GARLIC CAULIFLOWER 38
MASHED TURNIPS 40
ENSALADA TALONG – FILIPINO EGGPLANT SALAD 42
KETO MASHED POTATOES 44
BAKED CUCUMBER CHIPS 46
SWEET AND SPICY TOFU 48
KETO BREAD ROLLS 50
COCONUT FLATBREAD 53
HEARTY SEED BREAD 57
KETO VEGAN FLAXSEED WRAPS 60

BAGEL FLAX CRACKERS 63
VEGAN FLAXSEED BISCUITS 65
KETO MICROWAVE BREAD 68
CAULIFLOWER PIZZA CRUST 71
KETO TORTILLA CHIPS 73
COCONUT FLOUR PIZZA CRUST 76
CHICKPEA SWEET POTATO STEW 79
CHICKEN TOMATO SOUP WITH ROSEMARY 81
VEGAN AFRICAN PEANUT STEW 83
WHITE BEAN SOUP 85
WILD RICE AND MUSHROOM SOUP 87
COCONUT CURRIED EGGPLANT 91
VEGETARIAN MEXICAN LASAGNA 93
VEGETARIAN BUFFALO DIP 95
SPICED ACORN SQUASH 97
POTLUCK BEANS 99
SLOW COOKING BAKED POTATOES 101
SLOW COOKER TACO BAKE 103
WHITE BEANS AND PORK SAUSAGES 105
SIDE DISH RECIPES...107
BUTTER-FRIED GREEN CABBAGE 107
ROASTED FENNEL AND SNOW PEA SALAD 111
BAKED MINI BELL PEPPERS 113
KETO CAULIFLOWER RICE 115
KETO CAULIFLOWER HASH BROWNS 117

OVEN-ROASTED BRUSSELS SPROUTS WITH PARMESAN CHEESE 119
ZUCCHINI FETTUCCINE 121
BROWNED BUTTER CAULIFLOWER MASH 123
CONCLUSION **126**

INTRODUCTION

Thank you for being here and choosing this amazing keto vegan recipes guide.

Here in this book I have tried to include the best keto vegan recipes, suitable for everyone.

With a little patience you will try them and you will tell me how delicious.

But let's not waste time, get your pots and pans and utensils ready, let's get into the kitchen and start right away

VEGAN RECIPES

CAULIFLOWER BIBIMBAP

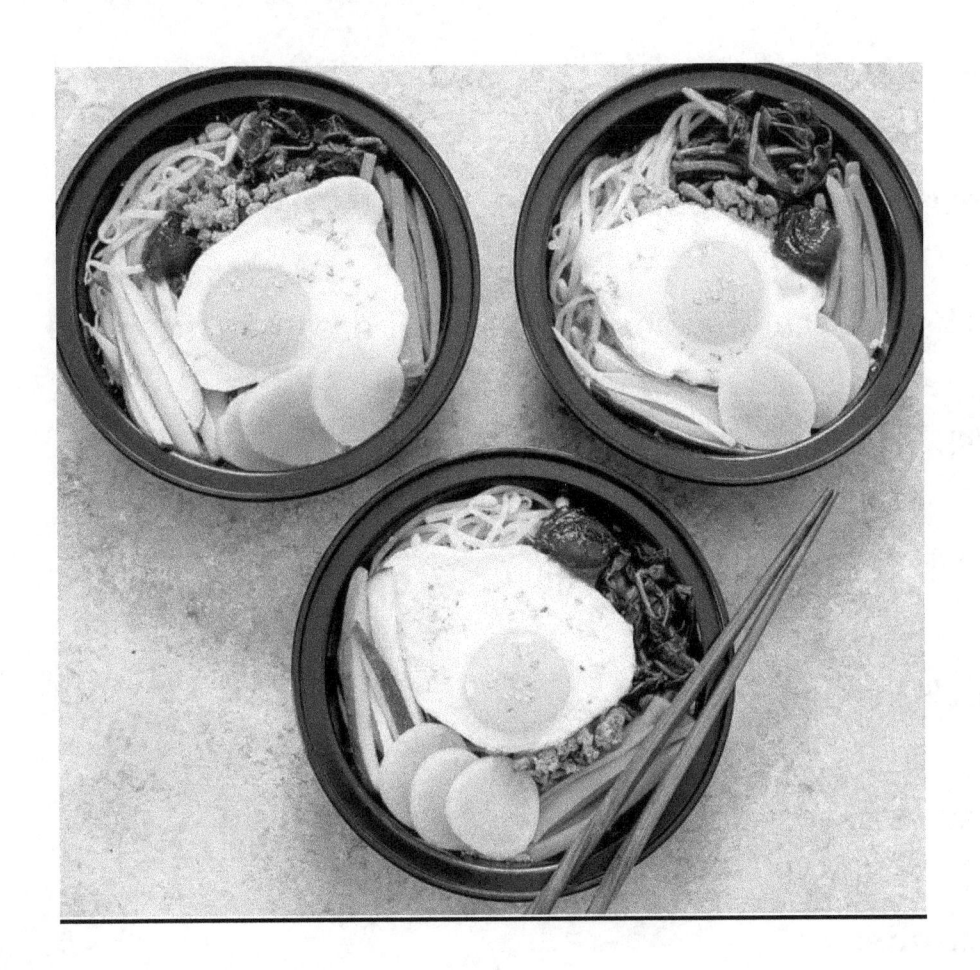

Ingredients

- 1 cup medium cauliflower

- 2 cups of kale

- 1 carrot peeled and cut into matches

- 6 oz sliced shiitake mushrooms

- 1 cup bean sprouts

- 2 cups fresh spinach

- 2 eggs

- 2 Tbsp low sodium soy gold sauce more, to taste

- 2 Tbsp sesame oil or more, to taste

- 2 Tbsp Sriracha sauce to taste

- Salt + pepper

- Sesame seeds (optional)

Instructions

1. For cauliflower rice: cut it into small pieces and place it in a food processor until it looks like grains of rice. For a large bowl, cover with a paper towel and microwave for 4 min

2. The boil has a pan of water. Add the bean springs and the bleach until they are slightly soft. Do not cook it too much.

3. Drain and place in a bowl. Add 1 Tbsp sriracha sauce, 1 tsp sesame oil, and 1 tsp sesame seeds and stir with the bean sprouts. Put aside.

4. Blanch the carrots in the same way and make sure you do not overcook them.

5. Brown the mushrooms in a medium with 1 Tbsp sesame oil until smooth. Add 1 Tbsp soy sauce to the fungus and place it on a plate.

6. Then cook the spinach in the kitchen and add a little soy sauce to season. Set aside spinach

7. Repeat the same process with kale

8. Fry the egg.

9. Stir in a bowl with cauliflower at the bottom, followed by vegetables and top with fried eggs.

Prep time: 15 min; **Servings:** 2

Macros: Cal 306 Fat 19g Saturated Fat 3g Cholesterol 163mg Carbs 23g Fiber 5g Sugar 7g Protein 14g

ROASTED BOK CHOY

Ingredients

- 1 large cup Bok choy
- ¼ cup avocado oil
- 1 tsp sea salt
- ½ tsp black pepper
- 4 cloves of garlic (minced)

Instructions

1. Preheat the oven to 425 F.
2. Cut the bok choy into quarters or eighths.
3. Place the bok choy in a single layer on a large baking sheet. Spray with 2 Tbsp avocado oil. Repeat the oil, salt, and pepper on the other side.
4. Spread chopped garlic through the bok choy with your hands.

5. Roast the bok choy for 10 min in the oven on the lower rack until the leaves begin to lightly char.

Prep time: 10 min; **Servings:** 4

Macros: Cal 152 Fat 14g Protein 3g Total Carbs 5g Net Carbs 3g Fiber 2g Sugar 2g

VEGAN SHAKSHUKA

Ingredients

- 2 Tbsp olive oil

- 1 8 g oFirm dry tofu

- 3 tsp harissa

- 1 Tbsp tomato puree

- 2 red bell peppers, cut into small cubes

- 1 tsp smoked pepper

- 1 large onion, diced

- 4 minced teeth

- 1 pinch of salt

- 1 tsp cumin

- 1 pinch of sugar

- 28 g of tomatoes, canned or freshly cut

- 2 tsp Za'atar grilled

- ½ cup labneh without sugar or vegan yogurt

Instructions

1. Cut the tofu in half lengthwise. Dry and cut them into cubes.

2. With olive oil, tomato puree, smoked pepper, harissa, onion, red peppers, garlic, sugar, cumin, and salt. Sauce until peppers are tender for 6-8 min Stir regularly.

3. Add the tomatoes and simmer for ten min until the vegetables. Place each cup or round tofu in the sauce, press the sauce is only visible, and the rest is immersed in the sauce. Let it simmer for ten min.

4. Throw the Za'atar up and serve with plain bread and Labneh.

Prep time: 10 min; **Servings:** 4

Macros: Cal 151, Carbs 15g, Fat 5g Protein 9g

REFRIGERATED VEGETABLE SALAD

Ingredients

- 1 lb of pickles or English cucumbers

- ½ medium onion, thinly sliced

- 2 Tbsp fresh dill packed

- 1 tsp sea salt

- Leave 1 tsp coconut sugar or more to taste for Whole30

- ¼ tsp ground black pepper was omitted for AIP

- 2 Tbsp apple cider vinegar

Instructions

1. Use a mandolin or sharp knife to cut the cucumbers into thin slices.

2. Place in a large bowl.

3. Add the remaining ingredients and mix gently.

Prep time: 5 min; **Servings:** 4

Macros: Cal 24 Sodium 586mg 25% Potassium 174mg 5% Carbs 4g 1% Fiber 1g 4% Sugar 2g 2%

GINGER, SESAME, WALNUT AND HEMP SEED LETTUCE WRAPS

Ingredients

Sauce:

- 2 Tbsp tamari
- 1 Tbsp maple syrup
- 1 tsp roasted sesame oil
- 2 Tbsp brown rice vinegar
- 1 Tbsp chopped ginger

Filling:

6. 1 cup chopped walnuts
7. ½ cup hemp seeds
8. 2 chopped dates
9. ½ cup chopped cucumber

10. ¼ cup chopped carrots

11. optional sesame seeds

Instructions

1. Mix the sauce ingredients.

2. Add chopped walnuts, hemp seeds, dates, cucumber, and carrots. Put in the fridge for at least 1 hour to mix the Ingredients.

3. Stack the mixture on the lettuce leaves. Cover with sesame seeds if desired.

Prep time: 10 min; **Servings:** 4

Macros: Cal 382 | Carbs 13 g | Protein 14 g | Fat 31 g | Saturated Fat 2g | Cholesterol 0 mg | Sodium 510 mg | Potassium 230 mg Fiber: 3 g | Sugar 6g | Vitamin A: 1465 IU | Vitamin C: 1.4 mg Calcium: 72 mg | Iron: 4.5 mg

ROASTED PEPPERS AND ONIONS

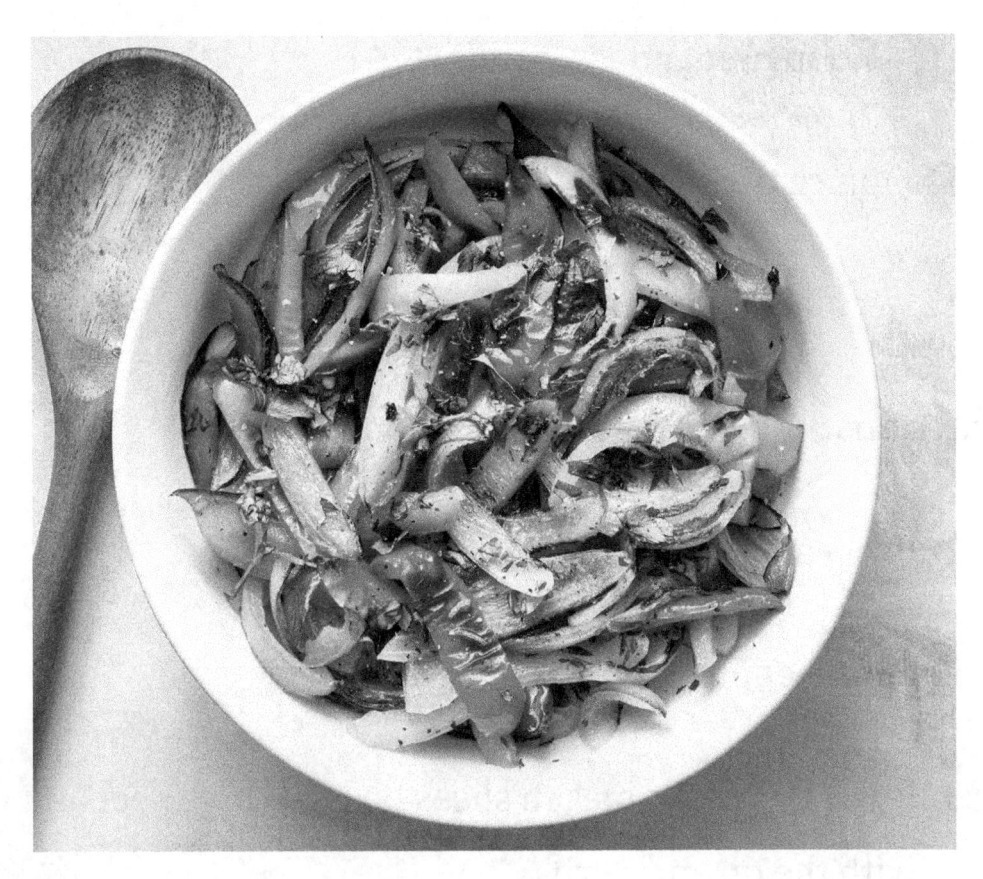

Ingredients

4. 1 red pepper

5. 1 orange pepper

6. 1 yellow pepper

7. 1 small onion

8. 1 tsp avocado oil

9. ½ tsp smoked pepper

10. ¼ tsp oregano

11. pinch of salt

12. A pinch of pepper

Instructions

1. Preheat oven to 400° F.

2. Chop peppers and onions.

3. Place the vegetables in slices on a baking sheet and mix with the oil and herbs.

4. Bake in 1 layer for 20 min

5. Stir after 20 min, then cook another 10 min if necessary.

Prep time: 5 min; **Servings:** 4

Macros: Cal 177 | Carbs 29 g | Protein 4g | Fat 5 g Sodium 15 mg Potassium 856 mg | Fiber 7 g | Sugar 13 g | Vitamin A: 8180°IU | Vitamin C: 527.5 mg | Calcium: 29 mg | Iron: 2 mg

CURRY PUMPKIN SOUP

Ingredients

- 13.5 g of coconut milk
- 15 g of pumpkin puree
- 2 Tbsp Thai red curry paste
- ¼ cup peanut butter
- ¼ cup water
- 2 tsp lime juice

Instructions

1. Put all the ingredients except the lime juice in a saucepan. Bring to a boil and simmer.
2. Boil until the peanut butter dissolves.
3. Add the juiced lime and serve.

Prep time: 5 min; **Servings:** 4

Macros: Cal 328 | Carbs 15 g | Protein 7g | Fat 29 g Saturated Fat 20 g | Cholesterol 0 mg | Sodium 92 mg Potassium 534 mg | Fiber 4 g | Sugar 5g | Vitamin A: 17725 IU | Vitamin C: 6.8 mg | Calcium: 62 mg | Iron: 5.1 mg

TOFU PERFECT BAKED CRISPY

Ingredients

- 1 extra stable tofu block

- ¼ cup Bragg Liquid Amino Acids Golden Soy or Tamari Sauce

- 1 Tbsp cornflour

Instructions

1. Drain the tofu: remove the tofu from the package and wrap the tofu block with paper towels. Carefully remove the excess moisture and set aside.

2. Preheat oven to 425 F and cover the baking sheet with parchment paper.

3. Once the tofu is drained, cut into cubes and place in a large bowl. Pour Bragg and sprinkle the cornflour on the tofu and stir gently until it is evenly covered, and the cornstarch is not dry.

4. Place the cubes on a sheet and cook for 25 to 30 min. Flip halfway through.

Prep time: 10 min; **Servings:** 4

Macros: Cal 98 Fat 5 g Saturated fat 1 g Carbs 2 g Protein 12 g

KETO CAULIFLOWER STUFFING

Ingredients

- 1 large cauliflower (cut into small flowers)

- 1 large onion (sliced)

- ¼ cup celery (chopped)

- 2 cloves of garlic (minced)

- ¼ cup olive oil (you can also use butter)

- ½ tsp bird spices

- ½ tsp dried thyme

- ½ tsp ground sage

- 1 tsp sea salt

- ¼ tsp black pepper

- 2 Tbsp fresh parsley (minced meat)

- ¼ cup nuts (minced pork)

Instructions

- Preheat oven to 450° F. Cover baking sheet with aluminum foil and grease well.

- Mix the chopped cauliflower, onions, celery, and garlic in a large bowl. Mix with olive oil, chicken herbs, sage, thyme, sea salt, and black pepper.

- Spread mixture in a single layer on the baking sheet. Roast in the oven for about 15 min, until the onions are tender and the cauliflower begins to brown. A little.

- Add the fresh parsley and nuts in the pan and mix everything. Roast again 10 to 15 min, until the pecans are lightly toasted, the cauliflower is golden brown, and the onions begin to caramelize.

Prep time: 10 min **Servings:** 4

Macros: Cal95 Fat7g Protein 2g Total Carbs 7g Net Carbs 4g Fiber 3g Sugar 3

KETO VEGAN PIZZA STICKS

Ingredients

- 1 extra stable tofu block

- ¼ cup + 1 Tbsp tomato sauce

- 2 Tbsp + 2 tsp nutritional yeast

- pinches of dried basil

Instructions

1. Drain the tofu: wrap a block of tofu in a paper towel. Place a cutting board on the tofu block. Press evenly on the top of the block by placing a cookbook on the cutting board. Drain the tofu for about 15-20 min

2. While the tofu is dripping, preheat the oven to 425 and cover the baking sheet with parchment paper.

3. Cut the tofu into 16 thin pieces and place them on a baking sheet.

4. Spread 1 tsp marinara sauce on each pizza bar.

5. Sprinkle ½ tsp nutritional yeast on each bar.

6. Sprinkle with basil on tofu sticks, to taste.

Prep time: 10 min; **Servings:** 4

Macros: Cal 133 Fat 6 g Saturated fat 1 g Sodium 21 mg Potassium 313 mg Carbs 7 g Fiber 3 g Protein 14 g

ZUCCHINI NOODLES WITH AVOCADO SAUCE

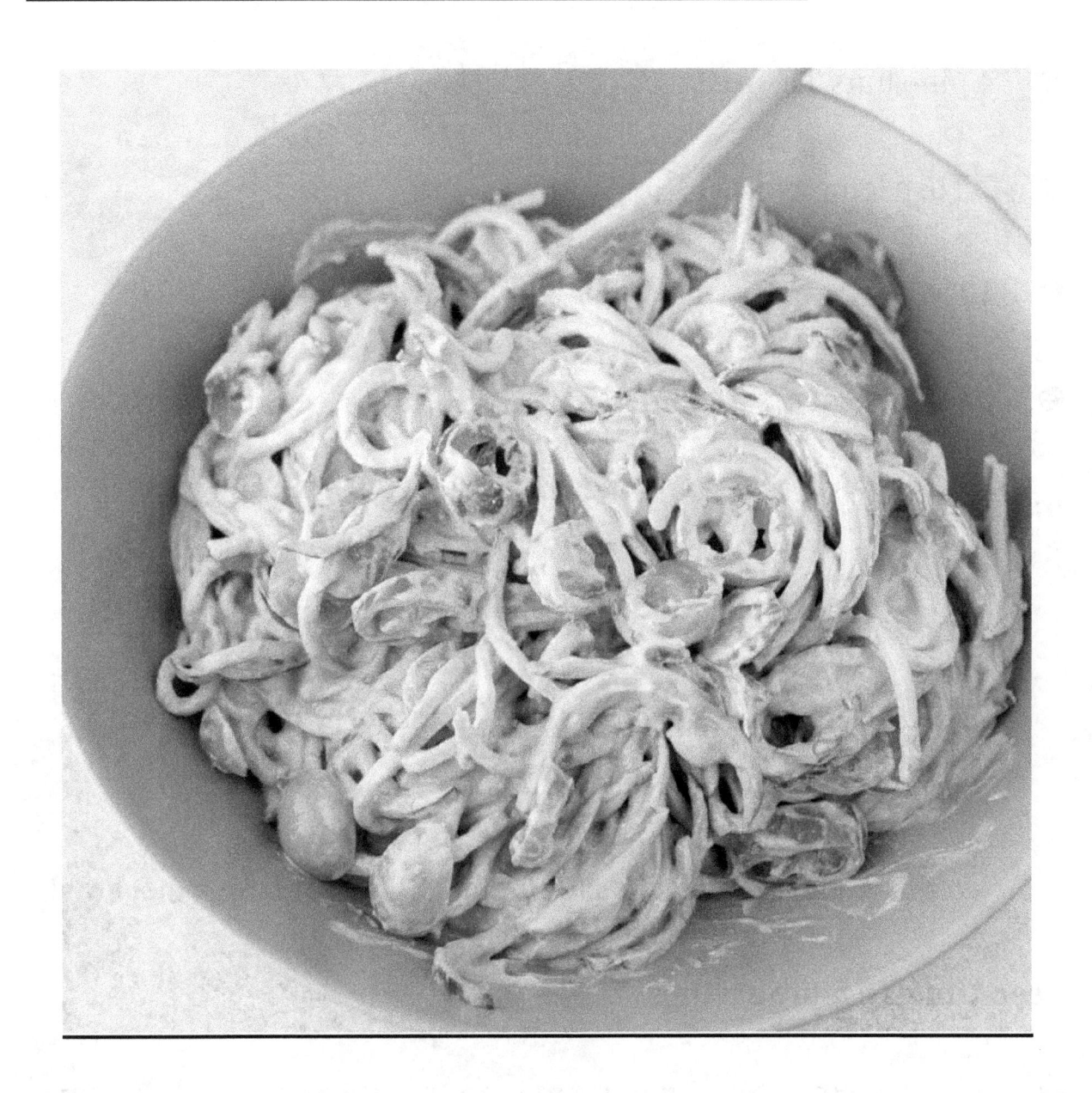

Ingredients

- 1 zucchini

- 1 ¼ cup basil (30 g)

- ⅓ cup water (85 ml)

- 4 pine nuts Tbsp

- 2 Tbsp lemon juice

- 1 lawyer

- 12 sliced cherry tomatoes

Instructions

1. Make zucchini noodles with a peeler or a spiralizer.

2. Mix remaining ingredients (except cherry tomatoes) in a blender until smooth.

3. Mix noodles, avocado sauce, and cherry tomatoes in a bowl.

Prep time: 10 min **Servings:** 2

Macros: Cal 313 Sugar 6.5 g Sodium 22 mg Fat 26.8 g saturated Fat 3.1 g Carbs 18.7 g Fiber 9.7 g Protein 6.8 g

VEGAN TOFU BUFFALO WINGS

Ingredients

- 1 block of extra firm organic tofu from House Foods
- ¼ cup hot sauce of your choice
- 1 Tbsp cornflour
- For an additional coating:
- ½ cup water
- 2 Tbsp hot sauce
- ½ tsp garlic powder
- ¼ tsp onion powder
- ¼ tsp pepper
- salt and pepper to taste
- 4 drops of Monk Fruit liquid Lakanto sweetener gold
- 8 drops of liquid stevia extract

- 1.5 tsp cornflour + 1 Tbsp water

Optional:

- Serve with a Vegan Ranch Vinaigrette

Instructions

1. Cut the drained tofu into 32 pieces of the same size and place in a large mixing bowl.

2. For the hot sauce, sprinkle the cornflour on the tofu and stir gently until it is evenly covered, and the cornstarch is not dry.

3. Heat a nonstick skillet over little heat (or sprinkle a nonstick skillet with an oil spray).

4. Cook the tofu for 3-4 min (until the bottom is golden), turn and cook the other side for another 3 min

5. While baking tofu, preheat oven to 425F, line a baking sheet with parchment paper and set aside.

6. Beat all additional Ingredients in a skillet and heat over medium heat. Let it thicken until it reaches the desired consistency (I did it 3 min), stirring occasionally. Put aside.

7. When the tofu is cooked, put it back in a large mixing bowl, add half the new coating mixture, and stir.

8. Place the tofu on a baking sheet and bake for 10 min on each side.

9. Remove from oven, cover with an additional coating. And serve with a Vegan Ranch salad dressing if desired.

Prep time: 10 min; **Servings:** 8

Macros: Cal 25 Fat 1 g 2% Sodium 219 mg Potassium 35 mg Carbs 1 g Protein 3 g

CAULIFLOWER RICE PILAF WITH HEMP SEED

Ingredients

- ½ cup cauliflower (2 cups of cauliflower rice)
- ½ cup hemp seeds
- 4 chopped dates
- ½ tsp turmeric
- ½ tsp cumin
- ½ cup low sodium vegetable broth
- ¼ cup sliced almonds
- Salt and pepper

Instructions

1. If you are using a cauliflower head, cut it into large pieces, and place it in the food processor. Mix until it looks like a rice consistency.

2. Chopped dates, turmeric, caraway, vegetable broth, and salt and pepper. Cook until liquid is absorbed, about 5 min

3. Add the sliced almonds.

Prep time: 5 min; **Servings:** 4

Macros: Cal 224 | Carbs 12 g | Protein 12 g | Fat 14 g Saturated Fat 1 g | Cholesterol 0 mg | Sodium 139 mg | Potassium 308 mg Fiber: 3 g | Sugar 6g | Vitamin A: 190 IU | Vitamin C: 34.7 mg | Calcium: 71 mg | Iron: 4.4 mg

GRILLED GARLIC CAULIFLOWER

Ingredients

- 1 medium cauliflower

- ¼ cup avocado oil (or light olive oil)

- ½ tsp sea salt

- ¼ tsp black pepper

- 4 garlic cloves, finely chopped

Instructions

1. Preheat the oven to 400° F. Grease a baking sheet.

2. Cut the cauliflower into ½ inch (1.25 cm) thick slices, then cut into small florets.

3. Mix the cauliflower in a large bowl with oil, salt sea, black pepper, and chopped garlic.

4. Place the cauliflower in a single layer on the baking sheet.

5. Bake for about 15-20 min, or until golden on the bottom. Turn over and cook another 5 to 10 min.

Prep time: 5 min **Servings:** 4

Macros: Cal161 Fat14g Protein 2g Total Carbs 8g Net Carbs 5g Fiber 3g Sugar 2g

MASHED TURNIPS

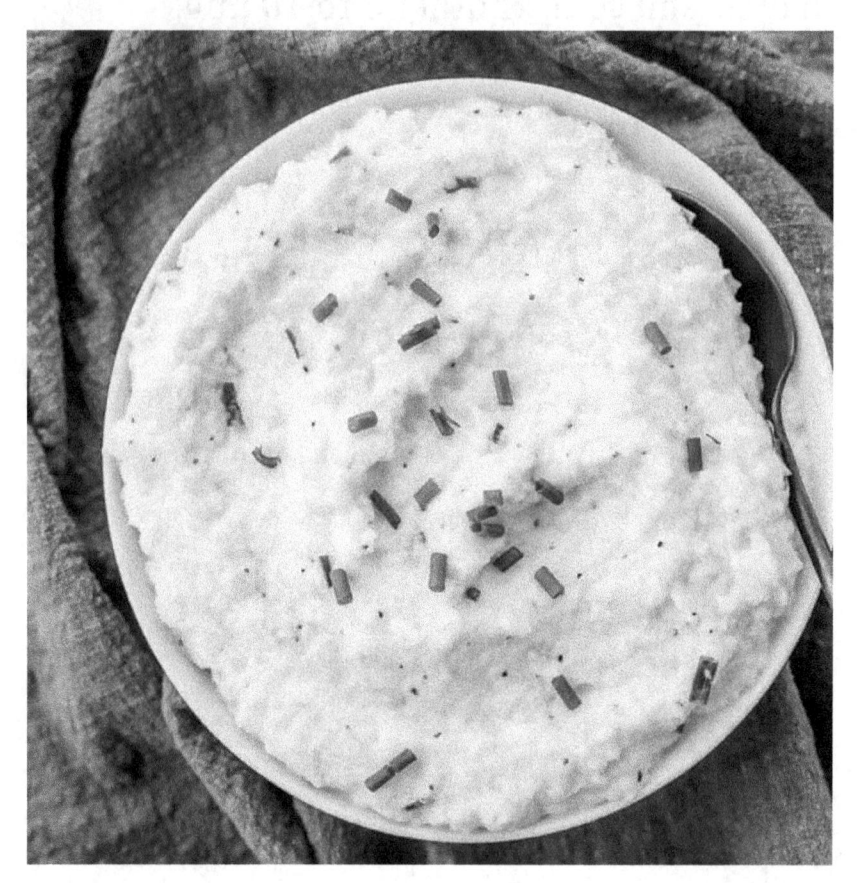

Ingredients

- ¼ cup coconut milk or almond milk

- 2 Tbsp coconut oil or butter with butter

- salt and ground black pepper to taste

- chives to decorate

- 1.5 lbs of turnips, peeled and quartered

Instructions

1. Cook the turnips in a saucepan until soft (about 30 to 45 min). Remove from water and place in a large bowl or food processor.

2. Add coconut oil with a taste of butter (or coconut milk) and almond milk (or ghee).

3. Mix with an electric mixer or food processor. Add low-carb milk if necessary. Add salt and pepper to taste.

Prep time: 10 min; **Servings:** 4

Macros: Cal 135 | Carbs 11 g | Protein 1g | Fat 10 g Saturated Fat 8 g | Cholesterol 0 mg | Sodium 115 mg Potassium 355 mg | Fiber 3g | Sugar 6g | Vitamin C: 35.7 mg | Calcium: 54 mg | Iron: 1 mg

ENSALADA TALONG – FILIPINO EGGPLANT SALAD

Ingredients

- 2 small eggplants
- 2 Tbsp apple cider vinegar
- 1 Tbsp white vinegar
- ½ tsp onion powder
- 1 tsp garlic powder
- salt and ground black pepper to taste
- roasted garlic garnished to garnish
- parsley to garnish

Instructions

1. Wash the eggplants well with cold water. Cut in half to open the eggplant and cut in pieces 1 to 2 centimeters long.

2. Using a baking sheet, place foil, and place the eggplant pieces down with the skin. Season with salt and pepper. Let stand 15 min wrap in aluminum foil.

3. Cook eggplant in an oven preheated to 400° For 10 to 15 min or until smooth. Let cool for 10 to 15 min,

4. After cooling, remove the skin and separate the eggplant into pieces with a fork.

5. Sprinkle onion and garlic powder and mix.

6. For apple cider vinegar and vinegar. Mix well.

7. Put in a bowl and cover with chopped garlic and wansoy.

Prep time: 35 min; **Servings:** 4

Macros: Servings: 1 cup | Cal 52 | Carbs 12 g | Protein 2g | Sodium 82 mg Potassium 415 mg | Fiber 7 g | Sugar 5g | Vitamin A: 100 IU | Vitamin C: 7.4 mg | Calcium: 20 mg Iron: 0.5 mg

KETO MASHED POTATOES

Ingredients

- 1 head of cauliflower (only florets, stems wholly removed)

- 3 cloves garlic (minced)

- 3 Tbsp butter (fixed size, then melted, you can also replace olive oil or ghee without dairy products)

- 1 Tbsp whole coconut milk (or thick cream for paleo)

- 3/4 tsp sea salt (adjust to taste)

- A pinch of black pepper (adjust to liking)

- 1 chopped Tbsp (finely chopped)

Instructions

8. Cook the cauliflower on the hotplate or in the microwave.

9. Stove Method: Boil a pan of water with a Tbsp (14 g) of salt. Add cauliflower and simmer gently (about 5-6 min). Drain well.

10. Microwave Method: Place the cauliflower flowers in a large bowl with 2 Tbsp water. Cover with plastic wrap so that the plastic does not touch the cauliflower. Microwave at high temperature for about 10 min, until they are very soft, Drain well.

11. Meanwhile, put the garlic, melted butter, and milk in a potent food processor or blender.

Prep time: 10 min; **Servings:** 4

Macros: Cal139 Fat10g Protein 4g Total Carbs 12g Net Carbs 7g Fiber5g Sugar5g

BAKED CUCUMBER CHIPS

Ingredients

- 2 medium cucumbers or 3 small

- 1 Tbsp olive oil or avocado

- 2 tsp apple cider vinegar or vinegar of your choice (leave aside for regular french fries)

- ½ tsp sea salt or more if needed

Instructions

5. Slice cucumber finely. For best results, use a mandolin cutter.

6. Remove excess moisture from the slices with a paper towel.

7. Put the cucumber slices in a large bowl and mix with the oil, vinegar, and salt.

8. For the dehydrator: place slices on trays and dry for 10-12 hours at 125-135 ° F or until crisp. For the oven: place the slices in a baking dish covered with parchment. Bake for 3-4 hours at 175 ° F or until crisp.

9. Let the slices cool before serving.

Prep time: 10 min; **Servings:** 6

Macros: Cal 25 | Carbs 1 g | Fat 2 g Monounsaturated Fat 2g | Sodium 396 mg | Potassium 51 mg | Vitamin A: 50 IU | Vitamin C: 0.8 mg

SWEET AND SPICY TOFU

Ingredients

4. 4 Tbsp vegetable oil

5. 200 g extra-strong tofu, drained and dry

6. 3 sliced new onions

7. 1 tsp minced garlic

8. ½ tsp chopped ginger

9. 2 Tbsp sriracha sauce

10. 2 Tbsp soy sauce

11. 1 Tbsp rice wine vinegar or balsamic vinegar

12. serf

13. 1 lime

14. 1 bunch fresh chopped mint

Instructions

48

1. Put the oil in a large saucepan and put on high heat.

2. In the meantime, make sure the excess liquid has been drained from your tofu block and cut into 1-inch cubes.

3. Add the rest of the tofu (you may need to cook in 2 portions, depending on the size of your pan) and cook for a few minutes before turning and frying on the other sides. They must be golden brown and crisp.

4. Once cooked, place it on a small cloth to wipe off the excess oil.

5. Keep the pan on the plate, but turn down on medium heat. Add the fresh onions, garlic, ginger, sriracha, soy sauce, and vinegar. Bake for a few min.

6. Put the tofu back in the pan and cover with sauce.

7. Sprinkle with chopped mint and a little lemon juice.

Servings: 2; **Prep time:** 10 min

Macros: Cal 60, Carbs 7g, Fat 2g Protein 5g

KETO BREAD ROLLS

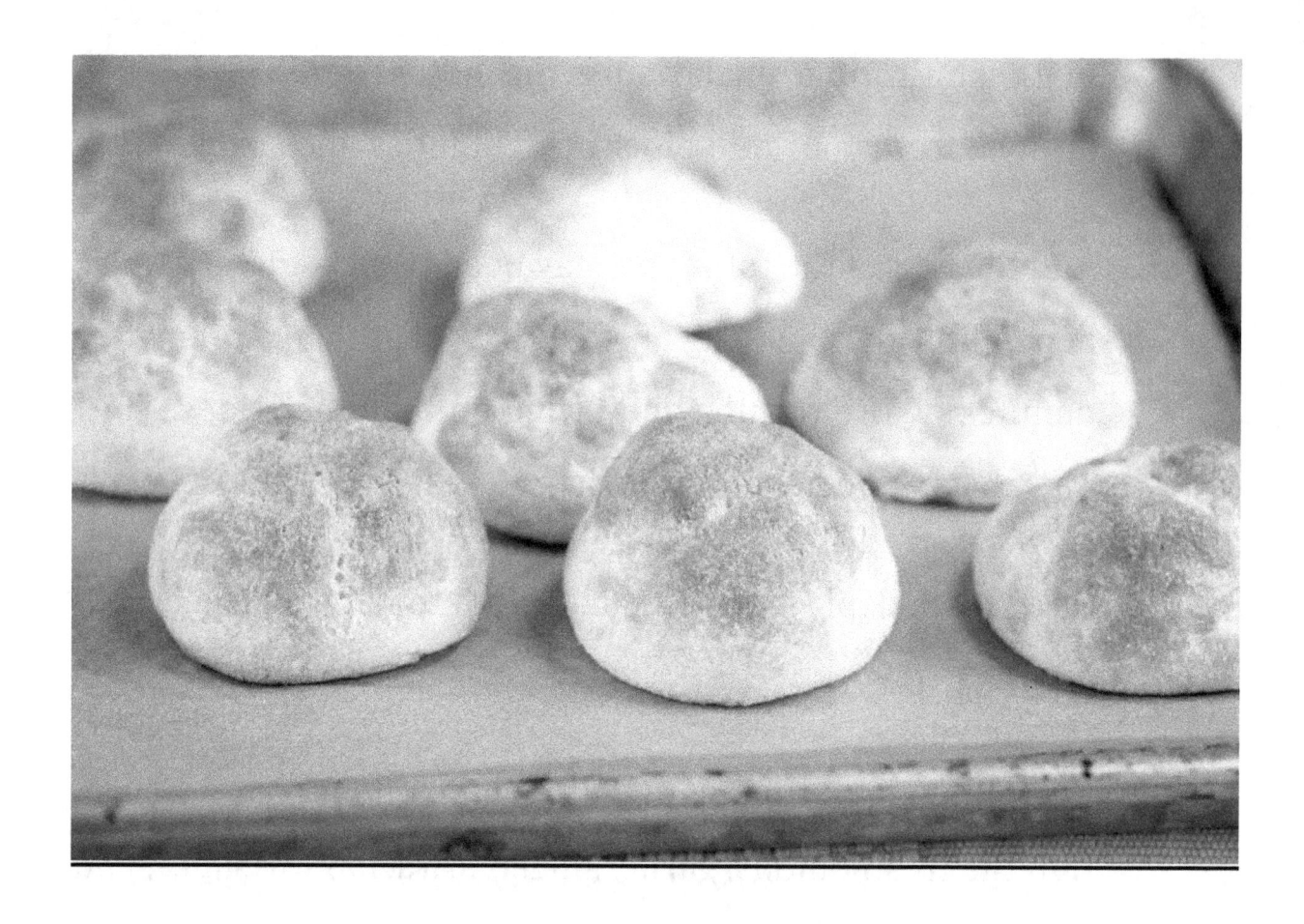

Ingredients

Dry Ingredients:

- 1 ¼ cups almond flour (150 g)

- ¼ cup coconut flour (30 g)

- ¼ cup + 3 Tbsp ground psyllium husk (37 g)

- ½ tsp salt

- 2 tsp yeast

Wet Ingredients:

- 2 tsp apple cider vinegar

- 1 Tbsp olive oil

- 1 cup hot water: 40 °C

- 2 Tbsp sesame seeds - optional

Instructions

1. Preheat the oven to 180°C. Prepare a baking sheet with parchment paper. Put aside.

2. In a large bowl, add all the dry ingredients: almond flour, coconut flour, ground psyllium peel, baking powder, and salt. Stir to combine.

3. Add apple cider vinegar, olive oil, and stir into hot water. Mix with a spatula for 1 minute; The water will be gradually absorbed, drying the mixture to make bread dough. It should

stay a little soft and sticky, which is normal but should be able to form a ball with your hand. If not, add a little more than 1 tsp zest at a time. If you want the ball to stay together, it's good when it's wet. Add no more than 1 Tbsp zest.

4. Wait 10 min for the fiber to absorb the liquid. The dough should be elastic, soft, and comfortable to be divided into 6 balls.

5. Roll each ball in your hands and place them on the baking sheet. It is not necessary to leave more than half an inch between each bread as they do not expand during cooking.

6. Brush the top of each loaf with a little tap water with a pastry brush.

7. Sprinkle sesame seeds on each bread, optional but delicious!

8. Cut half into slices and enjoy sandwiches with butter, ham, or cheese.

Prep time: 10 min

Macros: Cal 203 Fat 15 g Carbs 13.9 g Fiber 9.2 g Sugar 1.9 g Protein 6.2 g

COCONUT FLATBREAD

Ingredients

- 2 Tbsp psyllium skin (9 g)

- ½ cup excellent coconut flour, fresh, lump-free (60 g)

- 1 cup warm water (240 ml)

- 1 Tbsp olive oil (15 ml)

- ¼ tsp of baking powder

- ¼ tsp salt – optional

- 1 tsp olive oil to rub/grease the pan nonstick

Instructions

1. Mix the psyllium peel and coconut flour in a medium bowl.

2. Add warm water, olive oil, and baking powder. Mix well with a spatula and knead the dough with your hands.

3. Knead 1 minute. The dough is moist and becomes softer and slightly as it progresses. It must connect quickly to form a paste. If not, sticky, add more zest, ½ tsp at a time, knead for 30 seconds.

4. Place in the bowl for 10 min,

5. Now the dough must be soft, elastic, and well held; it is ready to roll.

6. Cut the dough into 4 equal pieces, roll each piece into a small ball.

7. Place 1 of the dough balls between 2 pieces of parchment paper, press the ball firmly on the paper with the palm of your hand and start rolling.

8. Remove the first layer of parchment paper from flatbread. Use a lid to cut the flatbread.

Cooking in Tray without Sticks:

4. Nonstick pancake pan on medium / high heat, or a non-stick pan of your choice, the 1 you would use for your pancakes.

5. Add tsp olive oil or vegetable oil of your choice on a piece of paper towel. Rub on the surface of the pan to make sure it is lightly greased. Do not let drops of oil. Otherwise, the bread will be frying!

6. Return the flatbread to the hot pan and carefully remove the last piece of parchment paper.

7. Cook 2 to 3 minutes on the first side, turn with a spatula and cook another 1 to 2 min on the other side.

8. Cool the flatbread on a plate and use it as a side dish. I recommend olive oil, crushed garlic, and herbs before serving! (optional but tasty!)

9. Repeat the rolling and baking for the next 3 flatbreads. Rub the greased paper towel on the plate.

10. Store in the pantry in an airtight container or on a flat cover with plastic wrap to keep them soft for up to 3 days.

11. If you want to give them some crunchy heat in a hot oven on a baking tray for 1-2 min at 150 ° C.

Prep time: 25 min **Servings:** 8

Macros: Cal 66 Fats 3.3 g Carbs 7.3 g Fiber 4.7 G Sugar 2 G Protein 2 g

HEARTY SEED BREAD

Ingredients

- 1 ½ cups raw pumpkin seeds (divided)

- ½ cup psyllium leaves (whole)

- 1 cup raw sunflower seeds

- ½ cup flax seeds

- ½ cup chia seeds

- 1 tsp fine sea salt

- 1 Tbsp maple syrup or a pinch of stevia powder

- 3 Tbsp olive oil

- 1 ½ cups warm filtered water

Instructions

1. Preheat the oven to 350° F; cover a 1 lb loaf pan with parchment paper and set aside.

2. Squeeze 1 cup pumpkin seeds in a food processor or blender until finely chopped. It must have a consistency of moderately thick flour (as shown in the photos).

3. Mix pumpkin seed meal with remaining pumpkin seeds, psyllium husks, sunflower seeds, flax seeds, chia seeds, salt, and maple syrup (or stevia) in a large bowl.

4. Then add warm water and olive oil and mix until the dough forms.

5. Squeeze the dough in the pan with your hands and cook for 45 min

6. Remove the shape of the oven and remove the bread. Place the dough on a baking sheet for 15 min

7. The bread is ready when you touch it, and it rings hollow inside.

8. Cool completely and cut into 16 pieces.

9. Serve grilled.

Prep time: 10 min; **Servings:** 8

Macros: 2 g net Carbs, 6 g Fat, 8 g Fiber, 7 g protein

KETO VEGAN FLAXSEED WRAPS

Ingredients

- 1 cup flaxseed

- 1 cup boiled water

- ½ tsp salt

- ¼ tsp turmeric

- ¼ tsp ground ginger

- ¼ tsp garlic powder

- ¼ tsp onion flakes

Instructions

8. Add flax seeds to a blender, mix on high speed until it forms a grind/meal. You can also use a Flax meal from the store, but make sure the flour is fine like almond flour, otherwise, it will not absorb all the water.

9. Boil the water in a small saucepan.

10. Remove from heat, add all the spices and add flaxseed all at once.

11. Stir with a wooden spoon until the food absorbs the water, dries and forms a ball of dough. As it moves, the mixture will form, which will gradually peel off the mold and form a ball of dough. It takes a maximum of 1-2 min

12. Remove the dough ball from the pan and place it on a piece of paper to prevent the dough from sticking to your work table. The mixture should not be maintained if it is. It means your food was not thin enough, and that's fine. Sprinkle extra food on the balloon to make it less sticky.

13. Divide the ball into 4 balls of the same size dough. Place another piece of baking paper on top of the dough from sticking to the roll. Lightly press the ball of dough with your hand and hold the parchment paper on the ball.

14. Roll with a rolling pin until it is flat, but not too thin or soft when cooked. Aim for a thickness of 2-3 mm. Remove the top piece of parchment paper.

15. Take a round shape like the lid of a pan, place it on the dough, and cut along the edges to make a circle.

16. Remove the lid and wrap the film on a nonstick skillet If you are not using a non-stick pan, sprinkle a little oil before putting the film in the pan.

17. Heat over medium heat and cook for 1 to 2 min or until the edge dries, the center is smooth, and you can quickly turn a spatula under the lid.

18. Cook about 1 more minute on the other side. Do not cook too much. It should be dry, but it remains soft to roll.

19. Place the cooked wrap on a plate.

20. Repeat these steps with the rest of the dough to form 4 rounds. You can reuse the same piece of parchment paper multiple times!

Prep time: 10 min

Macros: Cal 338 Fat 26.6g Carbs 18.5g Fiber 17.3G Sugar 1G Protein 11.6g

BAGEL FLAX CRACKERS

Ingredients

- 1 clove garlic minced

- 1 ½ cups of water

- 3/4 cup golden flaxseed

- ¼ cup brown flax seeds

- 3 tsp poppy seeds

- 3 tsp sesame seeds

- 3 tsp onion flakes

- 3 tsp garlic flakes

- 3 tsp sea salt

Instructions

1. Mix the garlic in the water in a blender or Nutribullet. For on the flax seeds. Soak for about 4 hours. The mixture becomes gelatinous.

2. Spread the mixture on a Teflon plate about 1/8 "to ¼" thick. Mark the mix with a knife and draw lines on the biscuits to make squares.

3. Mix all the herbs in a bowl, except the sea salt (it flows to the bottom of the pan). Sprinkle the whole mixture over the cookies. Then sprinkle with sea salt.

4. Dry at 110 ° for 24 hours or until crisp.

Prep time: 5 min; **Portions:** 6

Macros: Cal 44 Carbs 3 g Protein 1 g Fat 3 g Saturated Fat 0 g Cholesterol 0 mg Sodium 293 mg Potassium 74 mg Fiber 2 g Sugar 0 g Vitamin C: 0.5 mg Calcium: 27 mg iron: 0.5 mg

VEGAN FLAXSEED BISCUITS

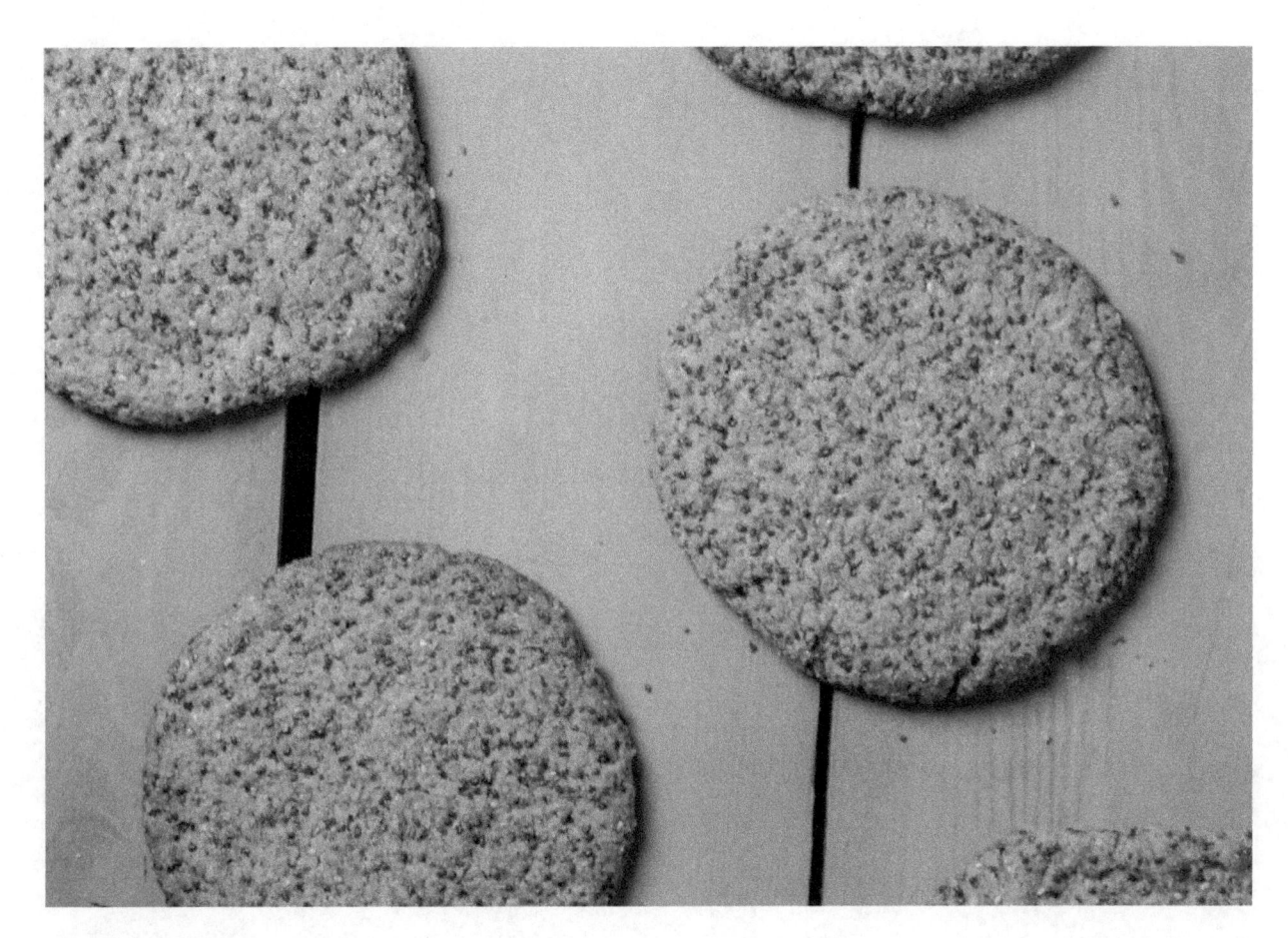

Ingredients

- 1 cup brown, golden ground flax seeds

- 2 tsp onion powder

- 1 tsp garlic powder

- ½ tsp salt

- 2 Tbsp black sesame - optional

- 2 white sesame Tbsp - optional

- 2 dried rosemary tsp

- ½ cup water

Instructions

1. In a mixing bowl, add ground flaxseed, onion powder, garlic powder, salt, sesame seeds, if available, and dried rosemary.

2. Mix well and for the water.

3. Use a spatula to mix all the ingredients at first, then use your hands to form a ball of dough. The more you knead, the drier the dough, the more dry and hard it becomes. If the ball really sticks to your hands, it can happen when your ground flaxseed is thicker than mine, sprinkle extra linseeds to lightly dry the ball, and make it easier to roll.

4. Place the ball of dough on 2 pieces of parchment paper and roll with a roll of about 2-4 mm thick. I love cookies!

5. Use a pizza cutter or knife to cut the rolled dough into squares/rectangles. I usually form a large box, then cut a small square out of it. I keep the remaining mixture from the edge to reform a ball, roll again and cut more biscuits with this paste. You must create a total of approximately 30 square cookies.

6. Leave the cookies on a piece of baking paper and slide the piece of paper on a baking sheet. Pierce each cookie 2-3 times with a fork.

7. Bake for 20-25 min at 350°F (180° C).

Prep time: 10 min; **Servings:** 4

Macros: Cal 38 Fat 3 g Sodium 81.6 mg Carbs 2.2 g Fiber 1.7 g Sugar 0.1 g Protein 1.3 g Calcium 30 mg IR 0.5 mg

KETO MICROWAVE BREAD

Ingredients

- ¼ cup flax flour
- 1 tsp coconut flour
- ¼ tsp of baking powder
- ½ tsp apple cider vinegar
- 1 Tbsp unsweetened almond milk

Seed mix:

- ¼ tsp sesame seeds
- ¼ tsp poppy seeds
- ¼ tsp pumpkin seeds
- ¼ tsp sunflower seeds

Instructions

1. In a small bowl, add flax flour, coconut flour, baking powder, cider vinegar, and unsweetened almond milk.

2. Use your hand to collect the ingredients and form a ball. It does not take more than a minute. The dough is a little sticky at first, but it turns quickly into a loaf of bread. On the contrary, if it is too dry, add a bit of almond milk ½ tsp at a time. This can happen if you use freshly ground flaxseeds, which are more pleasant and absorb more liquid.

3. Mix the seeds on a plate, place the ball of the bread on the seed, flatten the dough and stick the grain on 1 side. Repeat on the other side. You must finish with a 1 cm thick bread with seeds in both hands.

4. Place the bread on a plate, cook for 1 minute in a high-temperature microwave. You can add 30 seconds if you like your food as hard / hard as the French.

5. Remove from microwave and let cool 1 minute on a rack. The bottom of the bread is on the plate, it is healthy, it dries very quickly on the toaster.

6. Cut half of your bread and enjoy with your nut butter and sugar-free sweetener. Use the bagel mode and cook for 1 minute in height.

Prep time: 3 min; **Servings:** 5

Macros: Cal 141 Fat 10.1 g Carbs 8.3 g Fiber 7.1 G Sugar 0.5 g Protein 4.8 g 10%

CAULIFLOWER PIZZA CRUST

Ingredients

- 6 cups of cauliflower flowers 1 cup
- 1 cup ground flaxseed
- 2 tsp basil
- 2 tsp oregano
- ½ cup nutritional yeast
- 2 Tbsp olive oil + more to grease a baking sheet
- 1 tsp onion powder
- 1 tsp garlic powder
- salt and pepper

Instructions

4. Preheat the oven to 400° F.
5. Cauliflower steamed for 10-15 min Let cool.

6. Press as much water as possible into gauze or towel. This reduces the amount of cauliflower to about 3 cups.

7. Put the cauliflower and the rest of the ingredients in a food processor and mix well.

8. Spread ¼ of the Ingredients (on the size of your pizza) on a parchment paper. With slightly wet hands, spread the mixture about ¼ "thick, press firmly on the cauliflower.

9. Bake at 400° F for 20 min..

Prep time: 10 min; **Servings:** 4

Macros: Cal 340 | Carbs 22 g | Protein 13 g | Fat 24 g Saturated Fat 2g | Cholesterol 0 mg | Sodium 58 mg | Potassium 905 mg | Fiber 15 g | Sugar 3g | Vitamin A: 15 IU | Vitamin C: 72.5 mg | Calcium: 151 mg | Iron: 3.6 mg

KETO TORTILLA CHIPS

Ingredients

- 1 Tbsp black chia seeds

- ¼ cup water

- 1 cup almond flour

- 1 Tbsp olive oil

    4. ¼ tsp ground cumin

    5. ¼ tsp salt

    6. ¼ tsp garlic powder

    7. 1 tsp nutritional yeast

Instructions

1. Preheat the oven to 200 ° C.

2. Add the chia seeds and water in a small bowl. Stir with a spoon to combine. Allow to stand for 10 min or until a gelatinous texture is formed.

3. In another large bowl, add the almond flour, olive oil, spices, and chia seed

4. Knead the dough with your hands, squeezing the mixture between your fingers and the chia gel in the almond flour until it forms a paste. It does not take more than a minute to form a ball of dough.

5. Place the ball of dough between the 2 pieces of paper and unroll it with the most beautiful roll possible.

6. Remove the top layer of parchment paper, cut the tortillas with a pizza cutter or a sharp knife. To make triangular crisps (tortilla-shaped), simply place a round shape on the rolled dough. Cut around the lid, remove the dough from the cover, keep it turning again and make more fries! You should end up with a circle of rolled dough. A ring creates about 10 tokens, and you spin a total of 3 loops. Then cut the triangle with the pizza cutter as it cuts a round cake.

7. Move the dough with baking paper on a baking sheet.

8. Bake for 6 min, check the color, and stop cooking as soon as it turns golden brown. For thin chips, it took 6-7 min For thicker chips, it can take 8 to 9 min.

9. Remove from the oven until golden brown and let cool on the baking sheet for 5 min

10. Use a flat tool such as a knife or small spatula to remove/lift the tortillas from the parchment paper.

Prep time: 10 min;

Macros: Cal 20 Fat 1.5 g Carbs 0.8 g Fiber 0.4 G Sugar 0.1 G Protein 0.8 g

COCONUT FLOUR PIZZA CRUST

Ingredients

- ½ cup + 2 Tbsp coconut flour (75g)
- 2 Tbsp ground psyllium husk (9g)
- ¼ tsp salt
- 1 Tbsp extra virgin olive oil (15ml)
- 1 cup lukewarm water - not boiling, think bath temperature (240ml)

Instructions

1. Preheat the oven at 220° C (430F).

2. In a large bowl, add the coconut flour, psyllium peel, salt, olive oil, and warm water.

3. Combine first with a spatula or wooden spoon, then use your hand and knead the dough for 1 minute. The mixture will be very wet, and that's what you want. Collect the pieces of

dough and form a ball. If it is too dry, just add a little more water, 1 Tbsp at a time, until the mixture stays in place.

4. Place in the bowl for 10 min at room temperature.

Mass Rolls:

1. The ball of dough is firm, elastic, and ready to roll.

2. Lightly grease a sheet of parchment paper with olive oil.

3. Place the ball of dough in the middle of this sheet. Place another piece of paper on the balloon, press the balloon, and start rolling the roll until you reach the desired thickness. More pizza will be delicate and crispy!

4. Remember that it is crucial to roll the dough between the sheets of parchment paper. Otherwise, the dough will stick to your roll.

5. Remove the top sheet of parchment paper. Use a knife to cut a pretty circle of pizza or keep the shape you want. If you cut yours in a circle, use the dough from the edge to another pizza crust.

Coconut Pizza:

1. Your pizza base is now ready for cooking. Pull the sheet of parchment paper with the pizza base on a baking sheet and bake for 12-15 min

Pizza Base:

2. Remove from oven, tomato sauce spread, young spinach shoots, and grated mozzarella and olives do not hesitate to use the Ingredients

3. Return to oven for 5-8 min or until cheese is melted and grated. You can also turn on the oven for 1-2 min at the end of the cooking process.

Prep time: 15 min; **Servings:** 2

Macros: Cal 86 Fat 3.8 g Carbs 10.3 g Fiber 6.3 g Sugar 3G Protein 3 g

CHICKPEA SWEET POTATO STEW

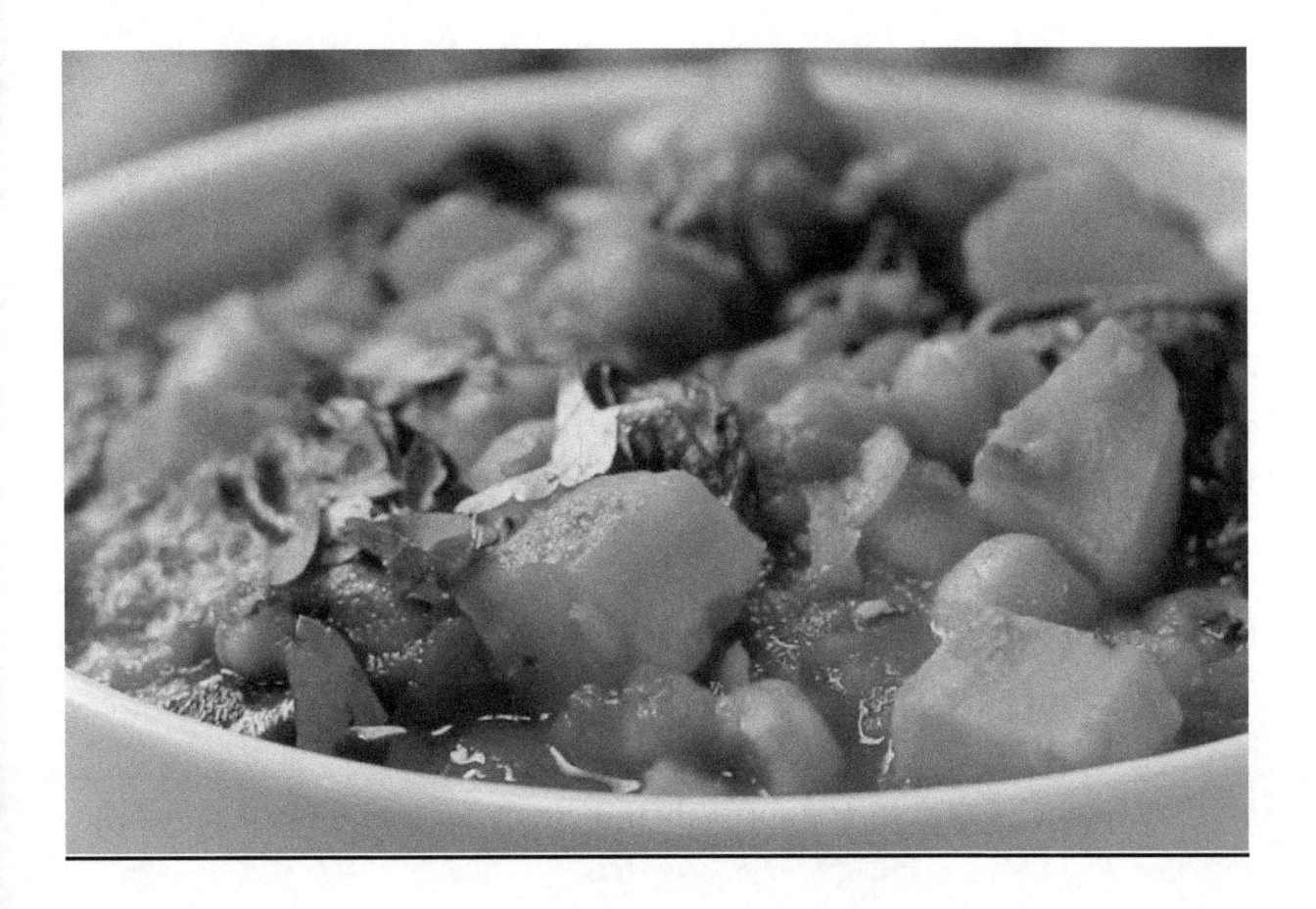

Ingredients

- A medium-sized yellow onion, chopped

- 2 cans of 15 oz chickpeas, drained

- 1 lb sweet potatoes, peeled and minced

- 1 Tbsp garlic, minced

- ½ tsp kosher salt

- ¼ tsp coarsely ground black pepper

- 1 tsp ground ginger, 1 ½ tsp ground cumin, 1 ground tsp coriander, ¼ tsp ground cinnamon

- 4 cups non-fat vegetable broth, 4 cups fresh spinach

Instructions

4. Except for spinach, add the Ingredients and cook for 8 min under high pressure.

5. Quick-release, for spinach and cover for 2 min until they fade.

Prep time: 15 min; **Servings:** 6

Macros: Cal 165 , Carbs 32.3 g, Protein 6.3 g, Fat 2.2 g, Saturated Fat 1.4 g, Sodium 751 mg, Fiber 6.2 g, Sugar 5.4 g

CHICKEN TOMATO SOUP WITH ROSEMARY

Ingredients

- 1 tsp olive oil, ½ cup chopped onion

- ½ cup chopped carrot, ½ cup diced celery, 2 garlic cloves, finely chopped

- Boxes of 15 oz chickpeas, rinsed and drained, 28-oz cans of crushed tomatoes

- 3 cups of low-sodium chicken broth or veggie vegetable broth, a sprig oFresh rosemary, 2 bay leaves

- 2 Tbsp chopped fresh basil, fresh black pepper, 2 cups fresh spinach, ¼ cup grated parmesan, more optional for decoration

Instructions

9. Heat the oil in a large nonstick skillet. Add carrots, celery, onions, garlic, and cook for 6 to 8 min until tender and fragrant. Add the broth, onions, chickpeas, parmesan, and pepper to the pan. Add rosemary, basil, and bay leaves, cover and cook on low heat for 6 hours.

10. When done, add the spinach. Cut the bay leaves, a sprig of rosemary, and season to taste. Serve the soup in bowls and, if desired, cover with additional Parmesan cheese.

Prep time: 10 min; **Servings:** 4

Macros: 1½ cups, Cal 215, Carbs 36g, Protein 9g, Fat 3g, Fiber 6g, Sugar 6g

VEGAN AFRICAN PEANUT STEW

Ingredients

8. 15 oz can chickpeas (drained and rinsed)

9. 4 cups vegetable broth

10. ½ tsp salt, 1 tsp cumin, ½ tsp ground coriander, ¼ tsp cayenne pepper, a 15-oz box of diced tomatoes (including the juice)

11. 4-5 cups sweet potatoes (cut into 2-inch cubes, about 2 medium-sized sweet potatoes), ½ cup natural peanut butter (creamy or crispy)

12. 1 onion (diced), garlic cloves (minced), 1-inch ginger (finely grated)

13. 4 handfuls of spinach

Instructions

1. In a 6-liter slow cooker, combine all ingredients and simmer for 6 to 8 hours.

2. Remove and cook the spinach for 15 min

3. Crush the sweet potato until stew thickens.

Prep time: 15 min; **Servings:** 8

Macros: Portion: 1/8 lot | Cal 263 | Carbs 36 g | Protein 10 g | Fat 9 g Saturated Fat 1 g | Fiber 7 g | Sugar 9 g |

WHITE BEAN SOUP

Ingredients

- 2 cans (15 g) of white beans

- A big carrot, peeled and cut into small cubes

- ¼ cup celery, diced, ½ cup yellow onion, diced, 3 garlic cloves minced

- ½ tsp chopped red pepper, tsp dried rosemary, tsp dried thyme, tsp dried oregano

- 2 ½ cups low sodium vegetable broth, 1 can (14 oz) diced tomatoes, 3 cups kale, minced meat, ½ cup grated and low-fat Parmesan cheese

Instructions

1. Drain and rinse the white beans.

2. Add all ingredients in a slow cooker, except kale and parmesan cheese. Cover and cook for 4 hours at low temperature or 2 hours at high heat, add kale and lid, and

cook another 30 min at high temperature or until wilted. Serve in bowls with parmesan cheese. Serve and enjoy!

Prep time: 10 min; **Servings:** 6

Macros: Cal 238 Fat 4 g Saturated Fat 2 g Carbs 37 g Fiber 10 g Sugar 4 g Protein 16 g

WILD RICE AND MUSHROOM SOUP

Ingredients

- 1 large onion, cut in half and finely sliced, 4 cloves garlic, finely chopped

- 700 g mushrooms

- 150 ml dry white wine

- 400 ml hot vegetable broth

- 180° g mixed white and wild rice, 3 Tbsp cream

- Small bunch of fresh parsley, minced

- salt, black pepper

Instructions

1. Add the onion, garlic, and sliced mushrooms to the slow cooker and for the white wine. Bake for 2 ½ hours, stir and scratch the sides after the first hour if you can.

2. When vegetables are very soft, add vegetable broth and rice and mix well. Cook another 2 hours on high heat or until rice is thoroughly cooked.

3. Add the cream and fresh parsley and season to taste. Serve immediately.

Prep time: 10 min; **Servings:** 3

Macros: Cal 345 , Carbs 61.5 g, Protein 17.1 g, Fat 3.2 g, Saturated Fat 1.6 g, Fiber 6.2 g, Sugar 9.2 g

RATATOUILLE

Ingredients

7. 2 Tbsp coconut oil (or ghee)

8. Broad onion, ground beef, 6 cloves of garlic, ground beef, broad aubergine, ground beef, orange pepper, ground beef, oven summer squash/zucchini

9. 1 cup chopped grape tomatoes

10. 1 cup chopped fresh basil

11. 2 Tbsp tomato puree

12. 1 tsp dried oregano

13. 1 tsp ground pepper

14. ½ - 1 tsp sea salt

15. ¼ tsp chopped red pepper (optional)

Instructions

1. Cover and cook all ingredients except basil in a large slow cooker. Cook 3-4 hours at high temperature or 5-6 hours at low temperature. When the vegetables are softened, the ratatouille is ready.

2. Add fresh basil before serving.

Prep time: 20 min; **Servings:** 8

Macros: Cal 127 Sugar 9 g Fat 5 g Carbs 23 g Fiber 10 g Protein 5 g

COCONUT CURRIED EGGPLANT

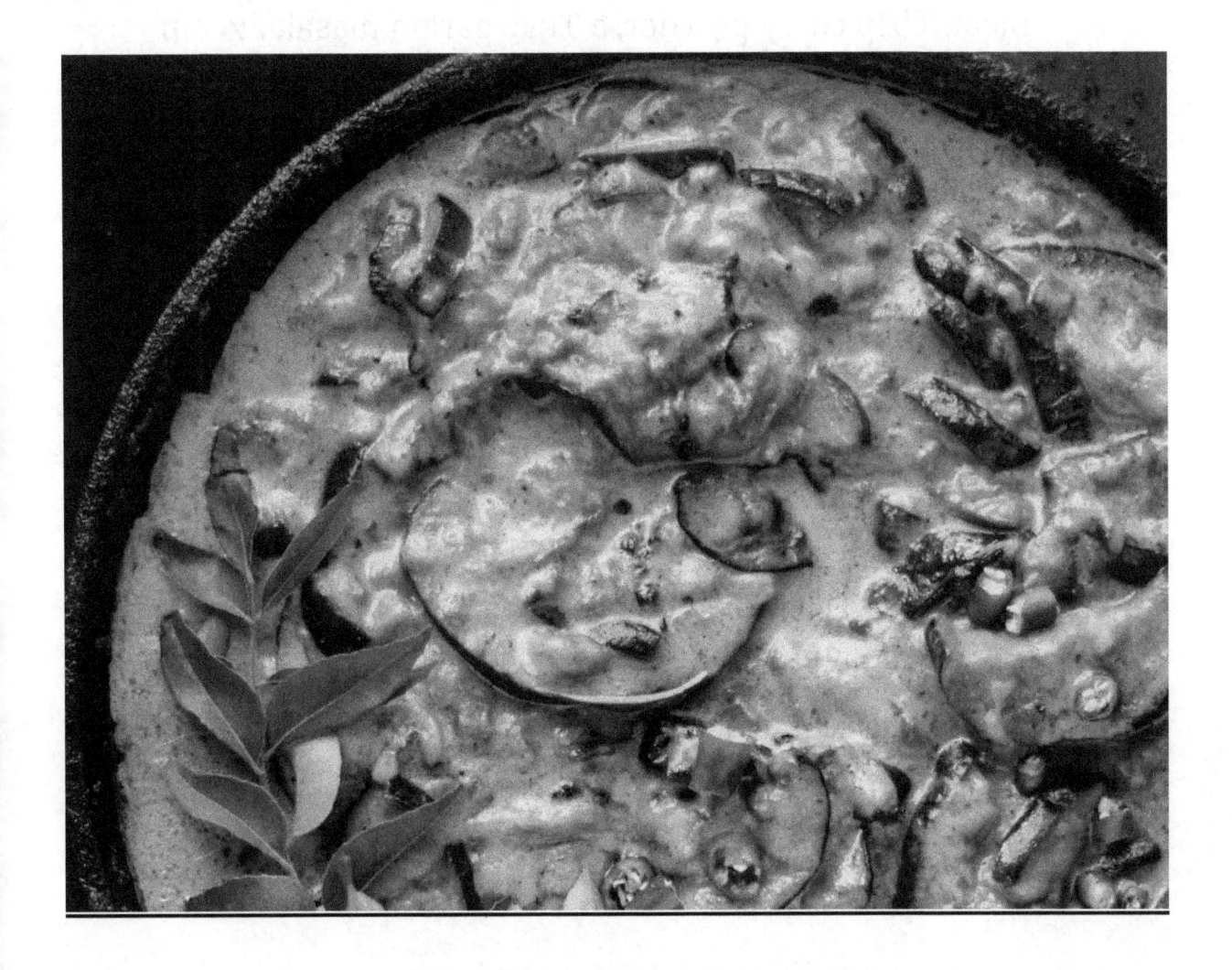

Ingredients

6. 4 cups minced eggplant (peeled, if desired)

7. 4 cups chopped zucchini, 6 oz tomato puree

8. 1 medium-sized yellow onion, 4 cloves of garlic, minced meat, Tbsp curry powder, a Tbsp garam masala, ¼ tsp cayenne pepper, ¼ spoon cumin, a tsp salt

9. Box of 15 oz coconut milk, ¼ cup vegetable broth (optional)

10. fresh parsley or chopped coriander to decorate

Instructions

5. Put the garlic and onion in a chopper to chop finely.

6. Add the chopped onion and garlic, eggplant, zucchini, herbs, tomato purée and coconut milk mixture to your slow cooker. Stir together. At this point, you can add vegetable broth. Simmer 4 to 5 hours.

7. Garnish with fresh parsley or coriander.

Prep time: 15 min; **Servings:** 4

Macros: Cal 321 Sugar 16 g Fat 24 g Carbs 27 g Fiber 5 g Protein 6 g

VEGETARIAN MEXICAN LASAGNA

Ingredients

- A box of tomato cubes with basil, oregano, and garlic

- 1 cup thick sauce

- 1 can (6 g) tomato puree

- ½ tsp ground cumin

- 2 boxes (15-1 / 2 oz each) of corn, rinsed and drained

- 1 can (15 g) unsalted black beans, rinsed and drained, 3 flour tortillas

- 2 cups grated Monterey Jack cheese.

- ¼ cup sliced ripe olives

Instructions

1. Split 3 25x3. High resistance aluminum bands; cross each other to appear as spokes of the wheel. Place the pieces in 5

quarters at the bottom and on the sides. Slow cooking Cover the slices with cooking spray.

2. Mix the tomatoes, sauce, tomatoes, and cumin in a large bowl. Place an omelet on the edge of the slow cooker. Cover with 1-third of the cheese and corn mixture. Repeat the layers twice. Sprinkle with olives: cover and cook for 3 ½ hours on low heat or until warm.

Prep time: 20; **Servings:** 8

Macros: 1 slice: 335 Cal, 12 g oFat (6 g of saturated fat), 41 g of Carbs (6 g of sugar, 8 g oFiber), 15 g of protein.

VEGETARIAN BUFFALO DIP

Ingredients

- 1 cup sour cream

- 8 g of cream cheese, softened, a mixture of ranch vinaigrette

- 2 cups shredded cheddar cheese;

- 1 can (15 g) of black beans, rinsed and drained

- 8 g oFresh mushrooms, minced meat

- Optional: sliced green onions and tortilla chips

Instructions

1. Mix the sour cream, cream cheese, and ranch dressing mixture in a bowl until smooth.

2. Add the following 4 Ingredients. Transfer to a 3 or 4 qt. slow cooker. Cook, covered, at high temperature for 1 ½ hours.

3. Sprinkle with green onions if desired and served with tortilla chips.

Prep time: 10 min; **Servings:** 6

Macros: ¼ cup: 113 Cal, 8 g fat (5 g of saturated fat), 21 mg of cholesterol, 526 mg of sodium, 5 g of Carbs (1 g of sugar, 1 g oFiber), 4 g of Protein

SPICED ACORN SQUASH

Ingredients

- 3/4 cup packed brown sugar

- tsp ground cinnamon

- tsp ground nutmeg

- 2 small pumpkins, cut in half and sown

- 3/4 cup grapes

- 4 Tbsp butter

- ½ cup water

Instructions

6. Add the brown sugar, cinnamon, and nutmeg in a small bowl; add half of the pumpkin. Sprinkle with grapes. Cover each butter with a cubic cupboard. Made of sturdy foil, cover each half separately and secure it.

7. Add water to a 5-liter slow cooker. Place the pumpkin on the side of the slow cooker (packages can be stacked). Cook over high heat for 3-1 / 2 to 4 hours, sealed or until pumpkin is tender. Open the sheet carefully so that the steam can escape.

Prep time: 15 min; **Servings:** 4

Macros: 433 Cal, 12 g fat (7 g of saturated fat), 31 mg of cholesterol, 142 mg of sodium, 86 g of Carbs (63 g of Sugar, 5 g oFiber), 3 g protein

POTLUCK BEANS

Ingredients

- 1 cup brewed coffee

- ½ cup brown sugar

- ¼ cup spicy brown mustard

- 2 Tbsp molasses

- 2 cans (16 g each) of butter beans

- 2 cans (16 g each) of red berries

- 2 cans (16 g each) of white beans

Instructions

9. In a greased 3 or 4 qt. Slow cooker, mix the first 4 ingredients. Rinse the beans and drain them; Stir in the coffee mixture. Bake in the sealed oven for 4 to 5 hours over low heat until flavors come together.

10. Freezing option: freeze-dried beans in freezer containers. To use, partially defrost in the refrigerator overnight. Heat in a covered pan, stir gently, and add a little water if necessary.

Prep time: 10 min; **Servings:** 12

Macros: ½ cup: 243 Cal, 0 Fat (0 saturated fat), 0 cholesterol, 538 mg of sodium, 50 g of Carbs (13 g of Sugar, 10 g oFiber), 14 g of protein.

SLOW COOKING BAKED POTATOES

Ingredients

- 6 medium brown, red potatoes

- 3 Tbsp soft butter, sour cream, butter, crumbled bacon, chopped chives

- 3 cloves of finely chopped garlic

- 1 cup water

- Salt and pepper to taste

- Guacamole, grated cheddar, chopped fresh coriander, optional

Instructions

1. Pierce the potatoes several times with a fork. Mix the butter and garlic in a small bowl. Rub the potatoes with the butter mixture. Wrap them tightly with a piece oFoil.

2. Add potatoes and water to slow cooker. Bake, cover, simmer for 8 to 10 hours or until tender. Season to taste and cover to taste.

Prep time: 10 min; **Servings:** 6

Macros: 1 potato: 217 Cal, 6 g oFat (4 g of saturated fat), 15 mg of cholesterol, 59 mg of sodium, 38 g of Carbs (2 g of sugar, 5 g oFiber), 5 g of Protein

SLOW COOKER TACO BAKE

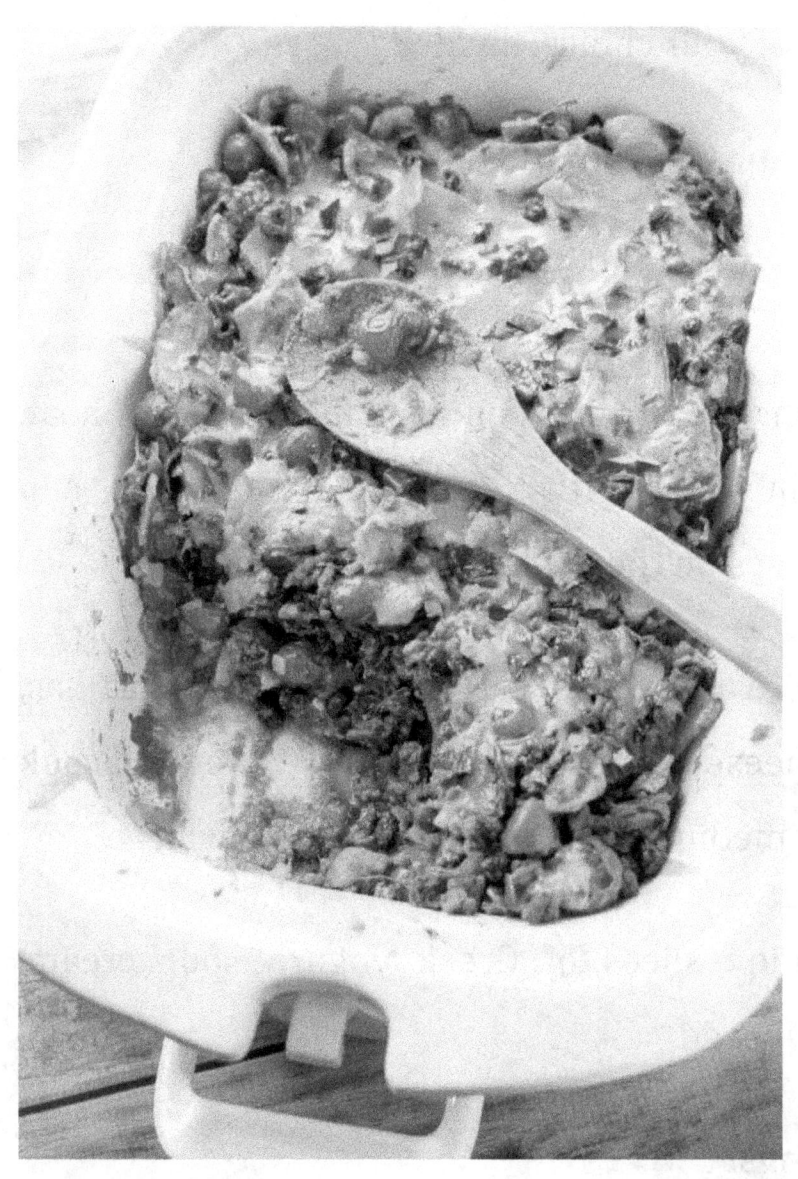

Ingredients

- A pack of gluten-free soft tacos Mission tortillas

- 1 lb lean ground chicken or turkey

- 1 can of 28 oz red enchilada sauce

- 1 cup grated cheese of your choice, divided

- 1 box of 4 g of black olives, divided

Instruction

4. Brown the ground in a frying pan over medium-high heat. Cut an omelet in strips with the enchilada sauce, ½ cup cheese and ½ olives on the golden meat. Shake to mix.

5. Add the mixture to a slow cooker. Cover with some tortillas, the rest of the cheese and olives on the tray; Cover and cook for 4 hours over medium heat or 8 hours over low heat.

6. If you wish, enjoy slices of Greek yogurt, sour cream, guacamole, or avocado.

Prep time: 5 min; **Servings:** 1

Macros: Cal 231, Fat 8g, Carbs 20g, Fiber 4g, Sugar 3g, Protein 20g

WHITE BEANS AND PORK SAUSAGES

Ingredients

- 4 cups of white beans

- 1 jar of crushed tomatoes

- 1 Tbsp garlic powder

- A Tbsp Celtic sea salt

- 12 g of kielbasa sausage

Instructions

1. Put the white beans in a large pan and cover with water. Let stand overnight at room temperature. Drain the beans for the next day.

2. Cover the seeds with water and add onions, garlic powder, salt, and sausage.

3. Place in saucepan, cover and cook for 8 hours or until the beans are tender. Add more salt or garlic powder to taste. Serve.

Prep time: 10 min; **For:** 8 people

Macros: Cal 2310.92 cal FAT 66.98 g Carriages 310.36 g Protein

SIDE DISH RECIPES

BUTTER-FRIED GREEN CABBAGE

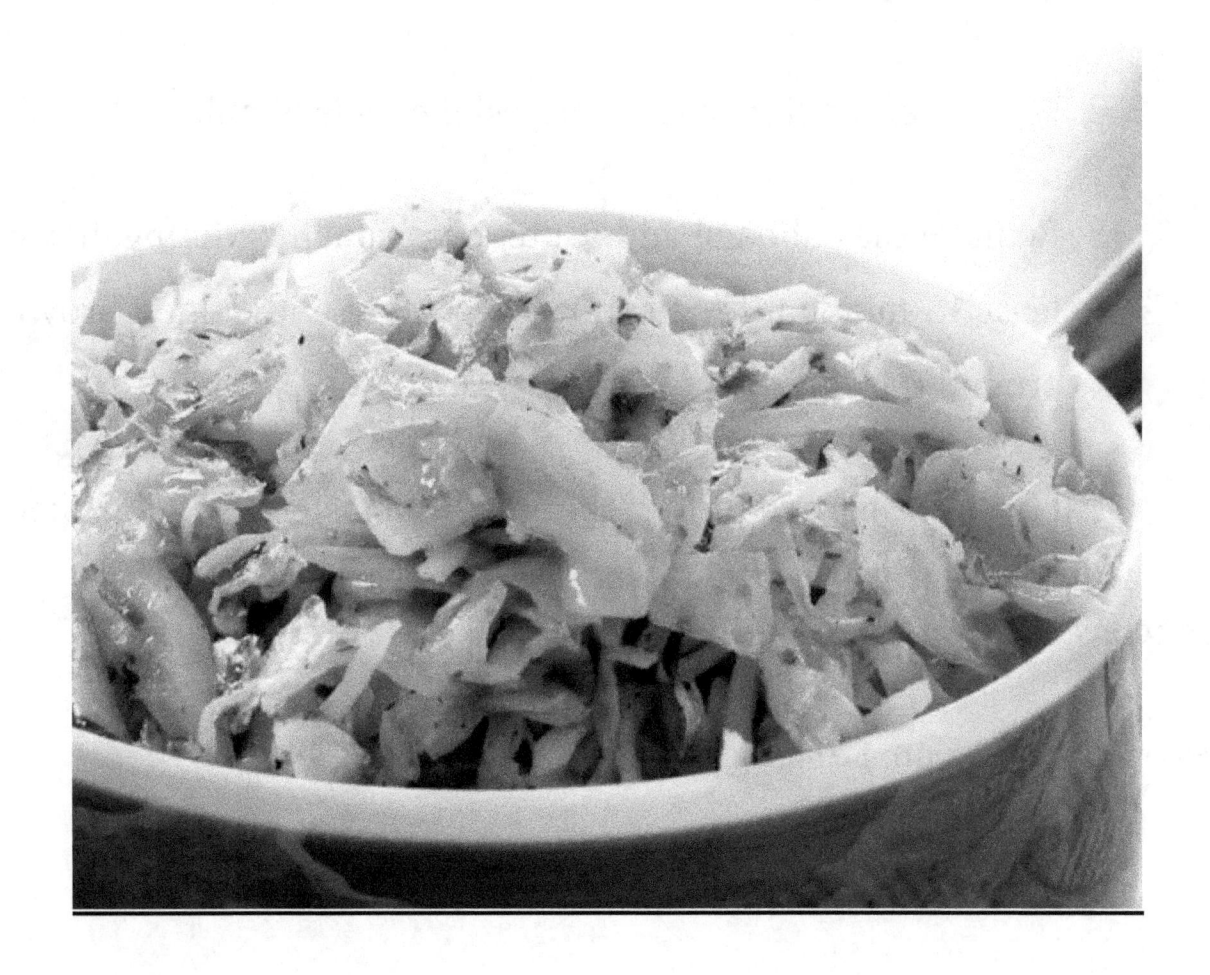

Ingredients

- 1½ lbs shredded green cabbage

- 3 oz unsalted butter

- salt and pepper

Instructions

1. Use a food processor, mandolin slicer, or a sharp knife to cut the cabbage.

2. Place over medium heat a large skillet. Stir in milk.

3. Remove the cabbage and sauté, occasionally stirring, for at least 15 min, until the cabbage is wilted and golden brown around the edges.

4. Lower the heat slightly to the edge— to taste salt and pepper.

Macros: Net Carbs (6 g), Fiber 4 g, Fat (17 g), Protein (2 g), 193

Prep time: 25 min; **Servings:** 4

COLESLAW

Ingredients

- ½ lb green cabbage

- ½ lemon, the juice

- 1 tsp salt, 1 Tbsp Dijon mustard

- 1/2 cup mayonnaise or vegan mayonnaise

- 1 pinch fennel seeds (optional), 1 pinch pepper

Instructions

1. Use a food processor, mandolin or sharp cheese slicer to cut the core and shred the cabbage.

2. Place the chicken in a bowl of medium size.

3. Add lemon juice and salt.

4. To allow the cabbage to wilt slightly, stir and let sit for 10 min Discard any liquid waste.

5. Mix the cabbage, mayonnaise, and mustard as an alternative.

6. Taste the season.

Macros: Net Carbs (3 g), Fiber 2 g, Fat (21 g), Protein (1 g), 209

Prep time: 15 min; **Servings:** 4

ROASTED FENNEL AND SNOW PEA SALAD

Ingredients

- 1 lb fresh fennel

- 3 Tbsp olive oil, sea salt

- 1 lemon, ground black pepper

- 2 Tbsp pumpkin seeds, toasted

- 5 oz snow peas

Instructions

1. Heat the oven to 225 ° C (450° ° F).

2. Cut off the fennel stalks and fronds. Then cut into small wedges, fennel bulb. Set aside in a baking dish. Add olive oil to the top. To taste salt and pepper.

3. Half the lemon and squeeze the juice out. Cut the lemon into thin wedges and then put it around the fennel.

4. Bake for 20–30 min in the oven or until a beautiful golden color has transformed into the fennel.

5. While baking the fennel, place the seeds of the pumpkin in a dry frying pan and toast for a few minutes over medium heat until browned but not burnt.

6. Mix the roasted fennel and the dry toasted pumpkin seeds with the raw shredded snow peas. Plate with fish, chicken or meat and serve.

Macros: Net Carbs (8 g) Fiber 5 g Fat (12 g) Protein (4 g) 165

Prep time: 40 min; **Servings:** 4

BAKED MINI BELL PEPPERS

Ingredients

- 8 oz mini bell peppers, about 2 per serving

- 1 oz air-dried chorizo, finely chopped

- 1 Tbsp fresh thyme, finely chopped or fresh cilantro

- 8 oz cream cheese, 4 oz shredded cheese

- ½ Tbsp mild chipotle paste, 2 Tbsp olive oil

Instructions

3. Set the oven at 200 ° C (325 ° F). Lengthwise break the peppers of the bell and remove the core.

4. Cut the chorizo and herbs perfect.

5. In a small bowl, combine the cream cheese, spices, and oil. Add the herbs and chorizo. Disable to smooth.

6. Fill the mixture with the bell peppers and put in a deep baking dish.

7. Sprinkle on top of shredded cheese. Bake for like 15–20 min until golden brown and the cheese is melted.

Macros: Net Carbs (6 g) Fiber 1 g Fat (37 g) Protein (12 g) 412

Prep time: 35 min; **Servings:** 4

KETO CAULIFLOWER RICE

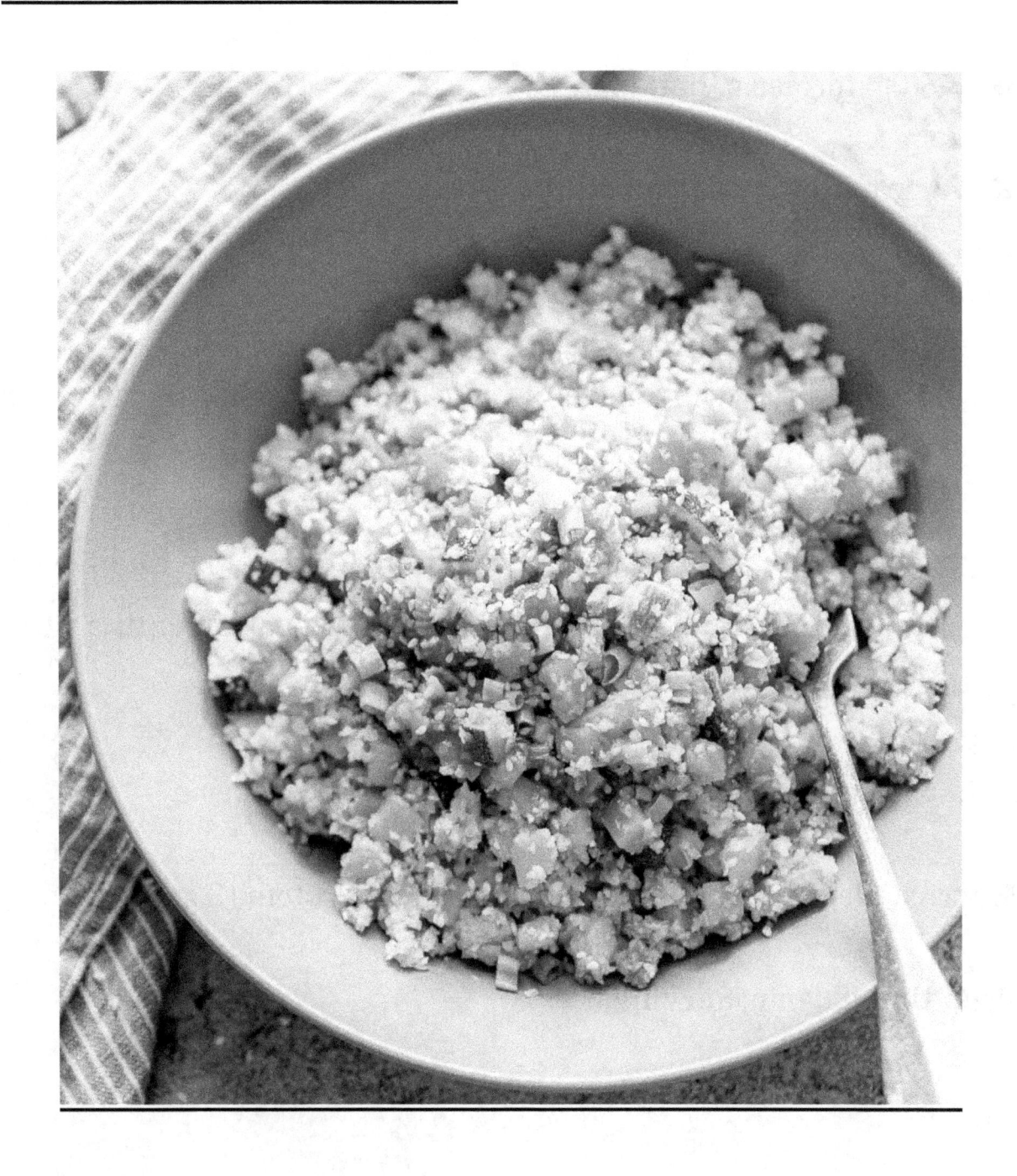

Ingredients

- 1½ lbs cauliflower

- ½ tsp salt

- ½ tsp turmeric (optional)

- 3 oz butter or coconut oil

Instructions

1. Shred the whole head of the cauliflower using a greater or grater Adamant on a food processor.

2. Melt in a pan butter or coconut oil. Remove the cauliflower and cook for 5-10 min over medium heat or until a little softened by the riced cauliflower.

3. During frying, add salt and the optional turmeric.

Macros: Net Carbs (5 g) Fiber 3 g Fat (18 g) Protein (3 g) 193

Prep time: 20 min; **Servings:** 4

KETO CAULIFLOWER HASH BROWNS

Ingredients

- 1 lb cauliflower

- 3 eggs

- ½ yellow onion, grated

- 1 tsp salt

- 2 pinches pepper

- 4 oz butter, for frying

Instructions

1. Use a food processor or grater to clean, cut, and grate the cauliflower.

2. Add a large bowl of cauliflower. Remove the rest of the ingredients and blend. Set 5–10 min aside.

3. Melt a generous quantity of butter or oil in a large skillet over medium heat. When you intend to have space for 3–4

pancakes (approximately 3-4 inches each) at a time, the cooking process will go faster. Use the low heat oven to keep the pancakes' first lots hot while you're making the others.

4. Place the rubbed cauliflower scoops in the frying pan and carefully flatten them until they are about 3-4 inches in diameter.

5. Fry on both sides for 4-5 min To make sure they don't burn, adjust the heat.

Macros: Net Carbs (5 g) Fiber 3 g Fat (26 g) Protein (7 g) 282

Prep time: 40 min; **Servings:** 4

OVEN-ROASTED BRUSSELS SPROUTS WITH PARMESAN CHEESE

Ingredients

- 1½ lbs Brussels sprouts
- 3 Tbsp olive oil
- 1 tsp dried rosemary or dried thyme
- salt and pepper
- 3 oz shaved parmesan cheese

Instructions

1. Heat the oven to 225 ° C (450° ° F).
2. Trim the sprouts from Brussels and cut them in half.
3. Layer in a baking dish and pour over the olive oil. Add rosemary/thyme and salt and pepper.

4. Roast for 15–20 min in the oven or until the sprouts in Brussels turned a beautiful color. Shave and enjoy parmesan cheese!

Macros: Net Carbs (9 g) Fiber 7 g Fat (16 g) Protein (13 g) 245

Prep time: 30 min; **Servings:** 4

ZUCCHINI FETTUCCINE

Ingredients

- 1 zucchini

- 1 oz olive oil or butter

- salt and pepper

Instructions

1. Prepare for approximately 1 zucchini of medium size per male.

2. Divide the zucchini lengthwise in half.

3. With a knife, scoop the seeds and cut the halves with a potato peeler rather thinly or use a spiralizer to make zoodles.

4. In a simmering sauce of your choosing, mix the zucchini noodles, and serve immediately.

5. If you don't use a sauce to eat your zucchini, boil half a gallon (a few liters) of salted water in a large pot and parboil the slices of zucchini for 1 minute.

6. Drain the water and stir and serve with olive oil or butter—salt and pepper.

Macros: Net Carbs 9 % (7 g) Fiber 3 g Fat 86 % (29 g)nProtein 5 % (4 g) 302

Prep time: 15 min; **Servings:** 1

BROWNED BUTTER CAULIFLOWER MASH

Ingredients

- 2 yellow onions, finely chopped

- 3 Tbsp butter, for frying

- 3 lbs cauliflower

- 1½ cups heavy whipping cream

- 10 oz shredded cheddar cheese

- 1 tsp sea salt

- ½ tsp ground black pepper

- 6 oz butter

Instructions

1. In a generous amount of butter, fry the chopped onions until soft and golden. Put it aside.

2. Shred the cauliflower with a grater's coarse side, or split it into smaller florets until it is rice-sized and chop in a food processor — filter at a time a few florets.

3. Pour heavy cream into a saucepan. Add the rice of the cauliflower and cook over medium heat. Let it cook for 10–15 min or more until the cauliflower is cooked thoroughly, and the cream is through. This will add a neutral flavor to the mash.

4. To taste salt and pepper. Add the onion fried and the cheese shredded. Mix well and stay warm.

5. Melt the butter for a soft, nutty taste at medium heat in a skillet until amber-colored. Serve the melted butter.

Macros: Net Carbs 7 % (10 g) Fiber 4 g Fat 83 % (49 g) Protein 10 % (13 g) 534

Prep time: 35; **Servings:** 8

CONCLUSION

Have you managed to conquer the woman or man of your dreams?

Have I succeeded with this cookbook to make you prepare wonderful dinners?

I have presented you with the best recipes, the tastiest and easiest to prepare, and now they are at your disposal.

Make good use of them, train every day and you will see the results.

Thank you for following me.

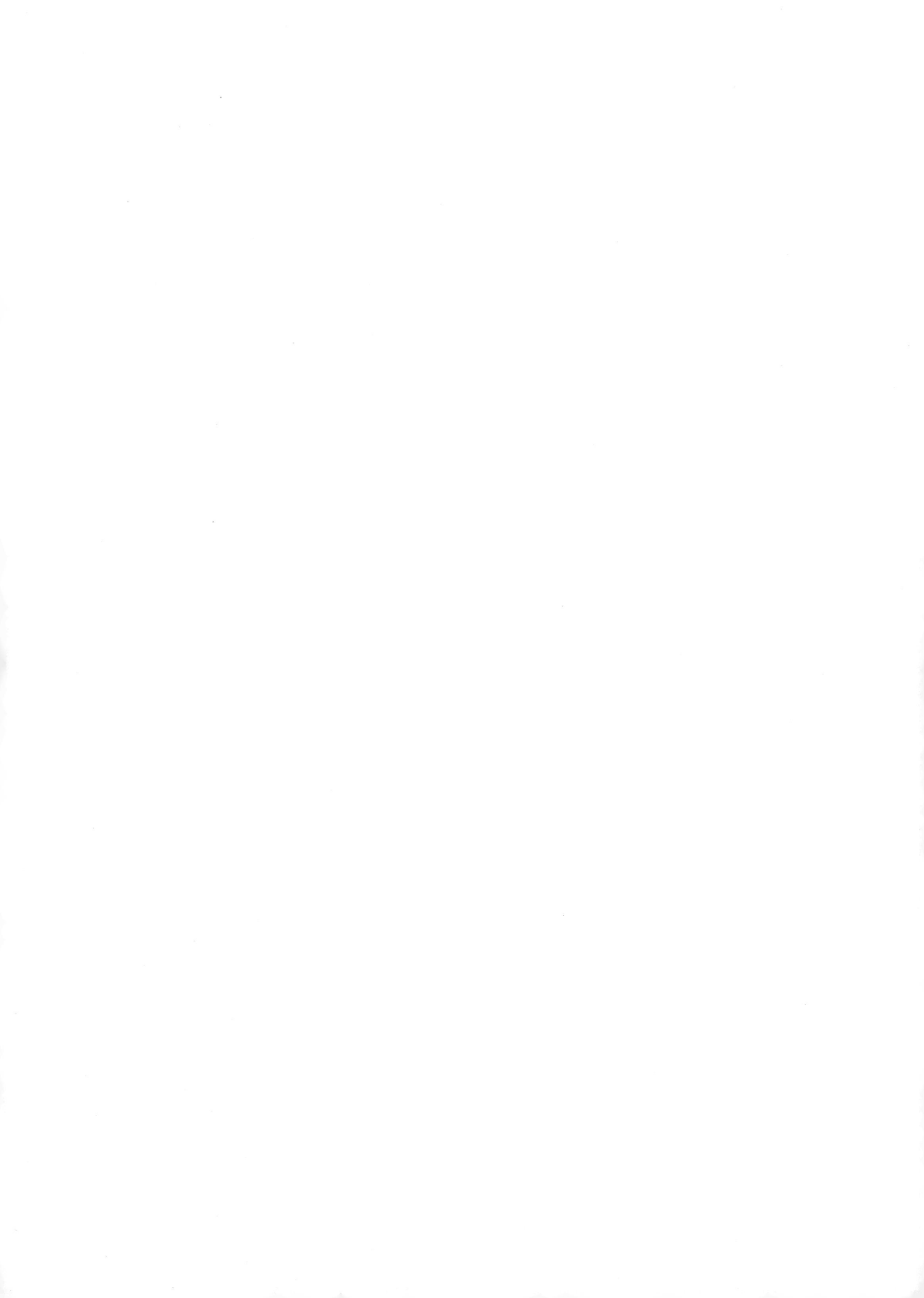